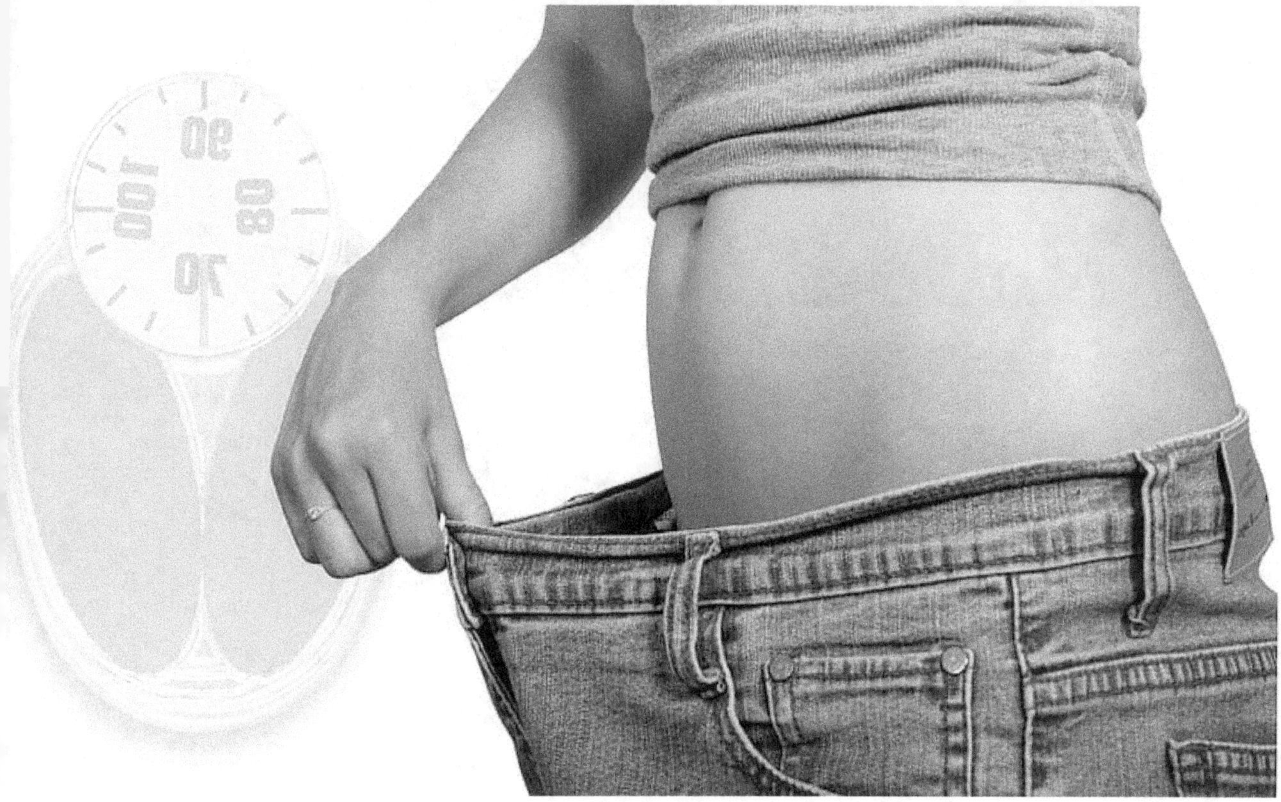

I0695520

Discover the Power of Natural Remedies for Effective Weight Loss

By Musodiq Akeusola

Table of Content

I. Introduction

- The challenges of weight loss
- The benefits of natural remedies

II. Green Tea Extract: Boost Your Metabolism and Burn Fat

- What is green tea extract?
- How green tea extract aids in weight loss
- Scientific evidence supporting the use of green tea extract for weight loss
- Recommended dosage and usage tips

III. Apple Cider Vinegar: Improve Digestion and Reduce Appetite

- Understanding apple cider vinegar
- How apple cider vinegar can help with weight loss
- Research on the effects of apple cider vinegar on weight loss
- Safe ways to consume apple cider vinegar for weight loss

IV. Garcinia Cambogia: Inhibit Fat Production and Suppress Appetite

- Introduction to Garcinia Cambogia
- How Garcinia Cambogia may assist with weight loss
- Scientific studies on Garcinia Cambogia and its effects on weight loss
- Considerations and precautions when using Garcinia Cambogia

V. Ginger: Boost Metabolism and Aid Digestion

- The properties of ginger for weight loss
- How ginger can help improve metabolism and digestion
- Evidence-based research on ginger for weight loss
- Different ways to incorporate ginger into your weight loss routine

VI. Cinnamon: Regulate Blood Sugar and Reduce Cravings

- Understanding the benefits of cinnamon
- How cinnamon can help regulate blood sugar and curb cravings
- Scientific studies on cinnamon and its effects on weight loss
- Recommended dosage and usage of cinnamon for weight loss

VII. Lemon Water: Detoxify and Hydrate for Weight Loss

- Lemon water as a natural weight loss remedy
- How lemon water can detoxify the body and support hydration
- Tips for incorporating lemon water into your weight loss routine

- Precautions and considerations when consuming lemon water

VIII. Additional Tips for Successful Weight Loss

- Importance of a balanced diet and regular exercise
- Incorporating healthy lifestyle habits for sustainable weight loss
- Managing stress and getting adequate sleep for optimal weight loss results
- Tracking progress and setting realistic goals for long-term success

IX. Safety Considerations and Precautions

- Consulting with a healthcare professional before starting any weight loss regimen, especially if you have any underlying health conditions or are taking medication
- Being aware of potential side effects or interactions of natural remedies
- Avoiding excessive or prolonged use of natural remedies without proper guidance
- Being mindful of individual allergies or sensitivities to specific natural remedies

X. Frequently Asked Questions (FAQs)

- Common questions related to using natural remedies for weight loss
- Providing evidence-based answers and clarifications on popular queries
- Addressing concerns and misconceptions about natural remedies for weight loss

XI. Success Stories and Testimonials

- Real-life experiences of individuals who have used natural remedies for weight loss
- Sharing inspiring success stories and testimonials to motivate and encourage readers
- Providing relatable examples of how natural remedies can be effective in achieving weight loss goals

XII. Conclusion

- Recap of the power of natural remedies for weight loss
- Emphasizing the importance of a holistic approach to weight loss that includes natural remedies, healthy lifestyle habits, and professional guidance
- Encouragement to explore and incorporate natural remedies for effective and sustainable weight loss

Introduction

Losing weight can be a challenging journey for many individuals. With numerous diets, supplements, and weight loss programs available in the market, it can be overwhelming to navigate through the options and find a safe and effective approach. However, in recent years, natural remedies have gained popularity as an alternative to support weight loss goals. Natural remedies for weight loss refer to various herbs, spices, extracts, and other plant-based products that are believed to aid in weight loss by promoting metabolism, reducing appetite, enhancing digestion, and supporting other physiological processes. These remedies are often considered safe and may offer additional health benefits beyond just weight loss.

In this article, we will explore the power of natural remedies for effective weight loss. We will delve into the scientific evidence supporting the use of specific natural remedies, their potential mechanisms of action, recommended dosages and usage tips, and safety considerations. It's important to note that while natural remedies can complement a healthy lifestyle and contribute to weight loss efforts, they should be used in consultation with a healthcare professional, especially if you have any underlying health conditions or are taking medication.

So, let's dive into the world of natural remedies and discover how they can be harnessed to support your weight loss journey in a safe and effective manner.

The challenges of weight loss

The challenges of weight loss are multifaceted and can vary from person to person. Many individuals struggle with losing weight due to various factors that may include:

1. Lifestyle habits: Unhealthy lifestyle habits, such as a sedentary lifestyle, poor diet choices, excessive consumption of processed or high-calorie foods, and irregular eating patterns, can contribute to weight gain and make weight loss challenging.
2. Emotional and psychological factors: Emotional eating, stress, anxiety, depression, and other psychological factors can affect eating behaviors and make it difficult to adhere to a healthy diet and

exercise routine, leading to weight gain or hindering weight loss efforts.

3. Genetics: Genetic factors can influence a person's metabolism, body composition, and fat storage patterns, making it harder for some individuals to lose weight despite their best efforts.

4. Medical conditions: Certain medical conditions, such as hormonal imbalances, thyroid disorders, polycystic ovary syndrome (PCOS), and other health conditions, can affect weight regulation and make weight loss more challenging.

5. Medication use: Some medications, such as corticosteroids, antidepressants, and antipsychotics, can cause weight gain or hinder weight loss efforts as a side effect.

6. Lack of motivation and consistency: Maintaining motivation, consistency, and adherence to a weight loss plan can be challenging, especially with busy lifestyles, social pressures, and other commitments that may hinder efforts to follow a healthy diet and exercise routine consistently.

7. Plateauing: Weight loss may initially occur at a faster rate but can slow down over time, leading to weight loss plateaus where the scale may not show progress despite efforts, which can be demotivating and challenging to overcome.

8. Unrealistic expectations: Unrealistic expectations about the rate of weight loss or aiming for an ideal body weight may lead to disappointment or frustration, making it challenging to stay committed to a weight loss plan.

9. Lack of support: Limited access to social support, such as friends, family, or a healthcare professional, can make weight loss challenging as it may be harder to stay motivated, stay on track, or seek guidance when needed.

In conclusion, weight loss can present various challenges that may differ from person to person. Addressing these challenges may require a holistic approach that involves healthy lifestyle changes, addressing emotional and psychological factors, seeking professional guidance when needed, and staying committed to a sustainable weight loss plan. It's important to remember that weight loss is a gradual and individualized process, and patience, consistency, and support are key factors in overcoming challenges and achieving long-term success.

The benefits of natural remedies

The use of natural remedies for weight loss can offer several benefits, including:

1. Safe and natural approach: Natural remedies typically use plant-based ingredients that are considered safe and have been used for centuries in traditional medicine. They are often free from harmful chemicals, artificial additives, and synthetic ingredients that may be present in some weight loss supplements or medications.
2. Improved overall health: Many natural remedies used for weight loss are rich in essential nutrients, vitamins, minerals, and antioxidants that can promote overall health. For example, herbs like green tea,

turmeric, and cinnamon are known for their antioxidant properties that can support cellular health and reduce inflammation.

3. Enhanced metabolism: Some natural remedies are believed to boost metabolism, which is the process by which the body converts food into energy. A faster metabolism can help burn more calories, resulting in increased weight loss. Ingredients like ginger, cayenne pepper, and black pepper are believed to have thermogenic properties that can boost metabolism.

4. Appetite suppression: Certain natural remedies, such as Garcinia Cambogia, green tea extract, and 5-HTP, are believed to help reduce appetite and curb cravings, which can aid in reducing overall calorie intake and supporting weight loss efforts.

5. Improved digestion: Many natural remedies are known to have digestive benefits. Ingredients like ginger, fennel, and peppermint can aid in digestion, reduce bloating, and improve gut health, which can indirectly support weight loss by promoting a healthy digestive system.

6. Flexibility and customization: Natural remedies offer a flexible and customizable approach to weight loss, as they can be incorporated into various forms such as teas, capsules, powders, or added to recipes. This allows individuals to tailor their weight loss plan according to their preferences and needs.

7. Cost-effective: Natural remedies can often be more cost-effective compared to some weight loss supplements or medications, as they are often readily available, affordable, and can be easily incorporated into a healthy diet and lifestyle.

8. Sustainable approach: Incorporating natural remedies into a healthy lifestyle can promote long-term sustainable weight loss habits. By focusing on natural remedies, individuals can develop healthy eating habits, regular exercise routines, and other positive lifestyle changes that can be maintained over the long term.

It's important to note that while natural remedies can offer potential benefits for weight loss, they are not a magic solution and should be used in conjunction with a healthy diet, regular exercise, and other lifestyle modifications for optimal results. It's always recommended to consult with a healthcare professional before starting any new weight loss regimen, especially if you have any underlying health conditions or are taking medication.

Green Tea Extract: Boost Your Metabolism and Burn Fat

Green tea extract is a popular natural remedy that has gained attention for its potential weight loss benefits. Green tea has been used for centuries in traditional medicine for its various health-promoting properties, including its ability to boost metabolism and burn fat. Here, we will explore the potential benefits of green tea extract for weight loss.

1. Metabolism Boost: Green tea extract contains catechins, which are natural antioxidants that are believed to help increase metabolism. Catechins, particularly epigallocatechin gallate (EGCG), have been shown to increase thermogenesis, which is the process by which the body produces heat and burns calories. This thermogenic effect can help increase metabolism and support weight loss efforts.
2. Fat Burning: Green tea extract is believed to help increase the breakdown of fat in the body, leading to increased fat oxidation. The catechins in green tea extract are known to inhibit the activity of an enzyme called catechol-O-methyltransferase (COMT), which is responsible for breaking down norepinephrine, a hormone that helps stimulate fat burning. By inhibiting COMT, green tea extract may help prolong the activity of norepinephrine, leading to increased fat burning.
3. Appetite Suppression: Green tea extract has also been suggested to help reduce appetite and curb cravings, which can aid in reducing overall calorie intake. The catechins in green tea extract are thought to help regulate ghrelin, a hormone that stimulates hunger, and increase the release of cholecystokinin (CCK), a hormone that promotes feelings of fullness. This can help individuals feel more

satiated and reduce their overall food intake, supporting weight loss efforts.

4. Antioxidant Properties: Green tea extract is rich in antioxidants, which can help neutralize harmful free radicals in the body and reduce oxidative stress. Oxidative stress can contribute to inflammation, cell damage, and other health issues that may hinder weight loss efforts. The antioxidant properties of green tea extract can help support overall health and well-being, which is important for maintaining a healthy weight.

5. Energy Boost: Green tea extract contains caffeine, a natural stimulant that can provide an energy boost. Increased energy levels can help individuals feel more motivated and engaged in physical activities, such as exercise, which is crucial for weight loss. However, it's important to note that the caffeine content in green tea extract may vary, and excessive caffeine intake may have adverse effects on health. It's essential to consume green tea extract and other caffeinated products in moderation.

6. Easy to Incorporate: Green tea extract is available in various forms, including capsules, tablets, powders, and teas, making it easy to incorporate into a daily routine. It can be consumed as a supplement or brewed as a tea, and can be a convenient addition to a healthy diet and lifestyle.

In conclusion, green tea extract has been studied for its potential benefits in boosting metabolism, burning fat, reducing appetite, and providing antioxidant properties, which can support weight loss efforts. However, it's important to remember that green tea extract is not a magic solution for weight loss and should be used in conjunction with a healthy diet, regular exercise, and other lifestyle modifications for optimal results. It's recommended to consult with a healthcare professional before starting any new weight loss regimen, especially if you have any underlying health conditions or are taking medication.

What is green tea extract?

Green tea extract is a concentrated form of the leaves of the Camellia sinensis plant, which is native to Asia and has been used for centuries for its various health benefits. Green tea extract is obtained by steeping the leaves of the green tea plant in a solvent, such as water or alcohol, to extract the bioactive compounds, including catechins, polyphenols, and other antioxidants that are believed to be responsible for its potential health-promoting effects.

Green tea extract is available in various forms, including capsules, tablets, powders, and teas. It is often marketed as a dietary supplement and is commonly used as a natural remedy for various health conditions, including weight loss, due to its potential thermogenic, fat-burning, appetite-suppressing, and antioxidant properties.

Green tea extract typically contains a higher concentration of bioactive compounds compared to brewed green tea, as it is made by extracting and concentrating the beneficial compounds from the tea leaves. The catechins in green tea extract, particularly epigallocatechin gallate (EGCG), are believed to be responsible for many of its potential health benefits, including its effects on metabolism, fat oxidation, appetite regulation, and antioxidant properties.

It's important to note that green tea extract is not a substitute for a healthy diet, regular exercise, and other lifestyle modifications for weight loss. It should be used in conjunction with a balanced diet and lifestyle for optimal results. As with any dietary supplement, it's recommended to consult with a healthcare professional before starting green tea extract or any other new supplement, especially if you have any underlying health conditions or are taking medication.

How green tea extract aids in weight loss

Green tea extract has been suggested to aid in weight loss due to its potential thermogenic, fat-burning, appetite-suppressing, and antioxidant properties. Here's how green tea extract may help with weight loss:

1. Boosts Metabolism: Green tea extract contains catechins, particularly epigallocatechin gallate (EGCG), which are believed to help increase metabolism. Catechins have been shown to increase thermogenesis, which is the process by which the body produces heat and burns calories. This thermogenic effect can help boost metabolism and increase calorie expenditure, potentially aiding in weight loss.

2. Enhances Fat Burning: Green tea extract is believed to help increase the breakdown of fat in the body, leading to increased fat oxidation. The catechins in green tea extract are known to inhibit the activity of an enzyme called catechol-O-methyltransferase (COMT), which is responsible for breaking down norepinephrine, a hormone that helps stimulate fat burning. By inhibiting COMT, green tea extract may help prolong the activity of norepinephrine, leading to increased fat burning.

3. Suppresses Appetite: Green tea extract has been suggested to help reduce appetite and curb cravings, which can aid in reducing overall calorie intake. The catechins in green tea extract are thought to help regulate ghrelin, a hormone that stimulates hunger, and increase the release of cholecystokinin (CCK), a hormone that promotes feelings of fullness. This can help individuals feel more satiated and reduce their overall food intake, supporting weight loss efforts.

4. Provides Antioxidant Properties: Green tea extract is rich in antioxidants, which can help neutralize harmful free radicals in the body and reduce oxidative stress. Oxidative stress can contribute to inflammation, cell damage, and other health issues that may hinder weight loss efforts. The antioxidant properties of green tea extract can help support overall health and well-being, which is important for maintaining a healthy weight.

5. Increases Energy Levels: Green tea extract contains caffeine, a natural stimulant that can provide an energy boost. Increased energy levels can help individuals feel more motivated and engaged in physical activities, such as exercise, which is crucial for weight loss. However, it's important to note that the caffeine content in green tea extract may vary, and excessive caffeine intake may have adverse

effects on health. It's essential to consume green tea extract and other caffeinated products in moderation.

It's important to note that the effects of green tea extract on weight loss may vary among individuals, and it is not a magic solution for weight loss. It should be used in conjunction with a healthy diet, regular exercise, and other lifestyle modifications for optimal results. As with any dietary supplement, it's recommended to consult with a healthcare professional before starting green tea extract or any other new supplement, especially if you have any underlying health conditions or are taking medication.

Scientific evidence supporting the use of green tea extract for weight loss The potential benefits of green tea extract for weight loss have been studied in numerous scientific research studies. Here are some scientific evidence supporting the use of green tea extract for weight loss:

1. Metabolic Effects: Several studies have shown that green tea extract can increase metabolism and energy expenditure. A meta-analysis of randomized controlled trials (RCTs) published in the American Journal of Clinical Nutrition in 2009 concluded that green tea extract significantly increased energy expenditure and fat oxidation, indicating its potential to boost metabolism and enhance fat burning.
2. Fat Oxidation: Green tea extract has been shown to increase the breakdown of fat in the body, leading to increased fat oxidation. A study published in the American Journal of Clinical Nutrition in 2008 found that green tea extract supplementation significantly increased fat oxidation during moderate-intensity exercise, suggesting that it may help the body use fat as a source of energy, which can aid in weight loss.
3. Appetite Suppression: Green tea extract has been suggested to help reduce appetite and curb cravings. A study published in the journal Obesity in 2009 found that green tea extract supplementation reduced self-reported hunger and increased satiety, leading to reduced food intake and lower calorie consumption. This suggests

that green tea extract may help regulate appetite and support weight loss efforts by reducing overall calorie intake.

4. Weight Loss: Several studies have shown that green tea extract can lead to modest weight loss. A meta-analysis of RCTs published in the International Journal of Obesity in 2009 concluded that green tea extract significantly reduced body weight and helped maintain weight loss, although the effects were modest. Another meta-analysis published in the Cochrane Database of Systematic Reviews in 2012 also found that green tea extract resulted in modest weight loss and was well-tolerated.

5. Antioxidant Properties: Green tea extract is rich in antioxidants, which can help reduce oxidative stress and inflammation in the body. A study published in the Journal of the American College of Nutrition in 2007 found that green tea extract supplementation significantly reduced markers of oxidative stress and inflammation, which can have positive effects on overall health and well-being, including weight management.

It's important to note that while these studies suggest potential benefits of green tea extract for weight loss, the results may vary among individuals, and it is not a substitute for a healthy diet, regular exercise, and other lifestyle modifications. As with any dietary supplement, it's recommended to consult with a healthcare professional before starting green tea extract or any other new supplement, especially if you have any underlying health conditions or are taking medication.

Recommended dosage and usage tips

The recommended dosage of green tea extract for weight loss can vary depending on the specific product, its concentration, and the individual's age, weight, and overall health. It's essential to follow the instructions on the product label or consult with a healthcare professional for personalized dosing recommendations. Here are some general dosage and usage tips for green tea extract:

1. Start with a low dose: If you're new to green tea extract, it's recommended to start with a low dose and gradually increase it as tolerated. This can help your body adjust to the extract and minimize the risk of potential side effects.
2. Follow the manufacturer's instructions: Different green tea extract products may have varying concentrations and dosages. Always follow the manufacturer's instructions and guidelines for the specific product you're using.
3. Consider caffeine content: Green tea extract naturally contains caffeine, which can have stimulant effects and may affect sleep, heart rate, and blood pressure. If you're sensitive to caffeine or have any health conditions that may be affected by caffeine, such as high blood pressure or cardiovascular issues, consider using a decaffeinated green tea extract or opting for a lower-caffeine product.
4. Take with food: Taking green tea extract with food can help minimize the risk of stomach upset and improve absorption. It's generally recommended to take green tea extract with a meal or a snack.
5. Stay hydrated: Green tea extract can have a diuretic effect and may increase urine production, so it's important to stay well-hydrated by drinking plenty of water throughout the day.
6. Monitor for side effects: While green tea extract is generally considered safe for most people, it can cause side effects in some individuals, including nausea, vomiting, stomach cramps, headache, and increased heart rate. If you experience any adverse effects, discontinue use and consult with a healthcare professional.
7. Combine with a healthy lifestyle: Green tea extract should not be considered a magic bullet for weight loss. It is most effective when combined with a healthy diet, regular exercise, and other lifestyle modifications, such as getting enough sleep, managing stress, and staying hydrated.

As always, it's crucial to consult with a healthcare professional, especially if you have any underlying health conditions, are pregnant or breastfeeding, or are taking medication, before starting any new dietary supplement, including green tea extract, to ensure it is safe and appropriate for your individual needs.

Apple Cider Vinegar: Improve Digestion and Reduce Appetite

Apple cider vinegar (ACV) has gained popularity as a natural remedy for weight loss due to its potential benefits in improving digestion and reducing appetite. ACV is a fermented liquid made from crushed apples, and it has been used for centuries for its purported health benefits. Here's what you need to know about how ACV may aid in weight loss:

1. Enhances digestion: ACV contains acetic acid, which has been shown to improve digestion by stimulating the production of digestive enzymes. Better digestion can help the body break down food more efficiently, absorb nutrients, and prevent digestive issues like bloating and constipation, which can impact weight management.
2. Reduces appetite: ACV has been suggested to help reduce appetite and increase feelings of fullness, which can potentially lead to lower calorie intake. Some studies suggest that ACV may help control blood sugar levels and delay gastric emptying, which can help regulate appetite and prevent overeating.
3. May increase metabolism: There is limited evidence to support the claim that ACV can directly boost metabolism. However, some studies suggest that acetic acid in ACV may improve the body's ability to burn fat for energy, which can potentially contribute to weight loss.
4. Supports gut health: ACV is believed to have prebiotic properties, which can help promote the growth of beneficial bacteria in the gut. A healthy gut microbiome has been linked to better digestion, metabolism, and weight management.
5. May help with insulin sensitivity: Some research suggests that ACV may help improve insulin sensitivity, which can be beneficial for individuals with insulin resistance or type 2 diabetes. Better insulin sensitivity can aid in blood sugar regulation and weight management.

6. Can be used in various ways: ACV can be consumed in different ways, such as diluted in water, used in salad dressings, or added to recipes. It's important to note that undiluted ACV can be harsh on the throat and teeth, so it's recommended to dilute it before consumption.
7. Considerations and precautions: ACV is highly acidic and may cause irritation or damage to the esophagus, tooth enamel, and digestive tract if consumed undiluted or in excessive amounts. It's crucial to use it in moderation and consult with a healthcare professional, especially if you have any underlying health conditions, such as acid reflux or kidney problems.

As with any natural remedy, it's important to use ACV as part of a comprehensive weight loss plan that includes a balanced diet, regular exercise, and other healthy lifestyle habits. It's also recommended to consult with a healthcare professional, particularly if you have any existing health conditions or are taking medications, to ensure that ACV is safe and appropriate for your individual needs.

Understanding Apple Cider Vinegar

Apple cider vinegar (ACV) is a type of vinegar that is made from fermented apples. It has been used for centuries for various health purposes and is believed to have numerous potential benefits. ACV is typically amber in color and has a strong, pungent smell and sour taste. It contains various bioactive compounds, including acetic acid, vitamins, minerals, enzymes, and beneficial bacteria.

ACV is known for its potential health benefits, including improving digestion, reducing appetite, supporting gut health, and potentially aiding in weight loss. It is also used for other purposes, such as a natural remedy for digestive issues, skin care, hair care, and household cleaning.

The process of making ACV involves fermenting crushed apples with the help of yeast and bacteria. The sugars in the apples are converted into alcohol through fermentation, and then further fermented into acetic acid, the main active ingredient in ACV. The acetic acid is responsible for the sour taste and many of the potential health benefits associated with ACV.

ACV is available in various forms, including raw, unfiltered ACV that contains the "mother," which is a cloudy, cobweb-like substance formed by the beneficial bacteria during fermentation. The "mother" is believed to contain beneficial enzymes, proteins, and probiotics that may contribute to the potential health benefits of ACV.

However, it's important to note that while ACV has been touted for its potential health benefits, scientific evidence supporting its effectiveness for specific health conditions, including weight loss, is limited and mixed. More research is needed to fully understand the mechanisms and effectiveness of ACV for weight loss and other health purposes.

When using ACV, it's essential to dilute it before consumption to avoid potential side effects, such as throat or digestive irritation. It's also crucial to use ACV as part of a balanced diet and healthy lifestyle, and to consult with a healthcare professional, particularly if you have any existing health conditions or are taking medications.

In conclusion, ACV is a popular natural remedy that has been associated with various health benefits, including potential weight loss effects. However, more research is needed to fully understand its effectiveness and safety. It's important to use ACV responsibly, as part of a comprehensive weight loss plan, and consult with a healthcare professional for personalized advice.

How apple cider vinegar can help with weight loss

Apple cider vinegar (ACV) has gained popularity as a potential natural remedy for weight loss. While scientific evidence is limited and mixed, some studies suggest that ACV may have certain properties that can support weight loss efforts. Here are some ways in which ACV may help with weight loss:

1. Appetite reduction: ACV has been found to potentially help reduce appetite. Acetic acid, the main active ingredient in ACV, has been shown to increase feelings of fullness and reduce overall calorie intake, which may help with weight loss efforts by reducing overeating or snacking between meals.
2. Improved digestion: ACV has been traditionally used to improve digestion, as it may help stimulate digestive enzymes and support gut health. A healthy digestive system is essential for optimal nutrient absorption and digestion, which can contribute to overall weight management.
3. Blood sugar control: ACV has been shown to potentially help regulate blood sugar levels by improving insulin sensitivity. Stable blood sugar levels can help prevent blood sugar spikes and crashes, which may impact hunger and cravings, ultimately supporting weight management.
4. Metabolism boost: Some studies suggest that ACV may help boost metabolism, which is the rate at which the body burns calories. A faster metabolism can aid in weight loss efforts by increasing calorie burning and energy expenditure.
5. Reduced fat accumulation: ACV has been found to potentially reduce the accumulation of fat in the body by inhibiting the conversion of sugars and starches into fat. This may help prevent excess fat storage, which can contribute to weight gain.
6. Support for healthy gut bacteria: ACV contains beneficial bacteria, enzymes, and probiotics that may promote a healthy gut microbiome. A balanced gut microbiome has been associated with various health benefits, including weight management.

It's important to note that while ACV may have potential benefits for weight loss, it's not a magic solution and should be used as part of a comprehensive weight loss plan that includes a balanced diet, regular exercise, and healthy lifestyle habits. ACV should be used with caution, as it can interact with certain medications and may cause side effects if used in excess or undiluted. It's recommended to consult with a healthcare professional before starting any new supplementation or weight loss regimen, especially if you have any existing health conditions.

Research on the Effects of Apple Cider Vinegar on Weight Loss

The potential effects of apple cider vinegar (ACV) on weight loss have been the subject of scientific research, although the evidence is limited and findings are mixed. Here are some key studies that have explored the effects of ACV on weight loss:

1. A study published in the Journal of Functional Foods in 2018 investigated the effects of ACV on body weight, body fat percentage, and waist circumference in overweight and obese individuals. The study found that participants who consumed 15 mL (about 1 tablespoon) of ACV daily for 12 weeks had significantly reduced body weight, body fat percentage, and waist circumference compared to the control group. The researchers concluded that ACV may have a beneficial effect on weight loss, but further research is needed to confirm these findings.
2. Another study published in the Journal of Clinical Nutrition in 2009 examined the effects of ACV on postprandial glycemia (blood sugar levels after a meal) and satiety in healthy individuals. The study found that consuming ACV with a high-carbohydrate meal resulted in lower blood sugar levels and increased feelings of fullness compared to a control group. The researchers concluded that ACV may help improve post-meal blood sugar control and reduce appetite, which could potentially aid in weight management.
3. A study published in the European Journal of Clinical Nutrition in 2018 investigated the effects of ACV on body weight, body fat, and appetite in healthy subjects. The study found that consuming ACV along with a high-carbohydrate meal resulted in increased satiety and reduced calorie intake compared to a control group. However, there

were no significant changes in body weight or body fat. The researchers suggested that ACV may have potential appetite-regulating effects, but further research is needed to determine its impact on weight loss.

4. A study published in the Journal of Medicinal Food in 2018 explored the effects of ACV on obesity-related parameters in high-fat diet-induced obese rats. The study found that rats fed a high-fat diet along with ACV supplementation had reduced body weight, body fat, and liver fat compared to the control group. The researchers concluded that ACV may help reduce obesity-related parameters in animals, but further research is needed to understand its effects in humans.

It's important to note that while some studies suggest potential benefits of ACV for weight loss, more research is needed to establish its effectiveness, optimal dosage, and long-term safety. It's also important to consider other factors such as individual differences, overall diet and lifestyle, and potential interactions with medications before incorporating ACV or any other supplement into a weight loss plan. Consulting with a healthcare professional or a registered dietitian is recommended for personalized advice.

Safe Ways to Consume Apple Cider Vinegar for Weight Loss

Apple cider vinegar (ACV) is a potent liquid that should be consumed with caution to ensure safety and effectiveness for weight loss. Here are some safe ways to consume ACV for weight loss:

1. Dilute with water: ACV is highly acidic and can potentially cause irritation or damage to the digestive tract, throat, and tooth enamel if consumed undiluted. It's essential to dilute ACV with water before consuming. Mix 1-2 tablespoons of ACV with 8-16 ounces of water to create a diluted solution.
2. Start with small amounts: If you're new to consuming ACV, start with small amounts and gradually increase the dosage over time. Begin

with 1 teaspoon of ACV in water and gradually work your way up to 1-2 tablespoons, depending on your tolerance and response.

3. Avoid excessive consumption: ACV is not meant to be consumed in large amounts. Excessive intake of ACV can lead to adverse effects such as digestive discomfort, low potassium levels, and tooth enamel erosion. Stick to recommended dosages and do not exceed the safe limits.

4. Take before meals: ACV may help with appetite regulation and blood sugar control, so it's commonly consumed before meals to potentially reduce appetite and aid in digestion. Take ACV 15-30 minutes before meals to potentially enhance its effects on weight loss.

5. Use quality, organic ACV: Choose a high-quality, organic, unfiltered, and unpasteurized ACV to ensure that you're getting the most benefits from its natural compounds. Look for brands that contain the "Mother" – a cloudy, sediment-like substance that contains beneficial enzymes and probiotics.

6. Consider other forms of consumption: If you find it challenging to tolerate the taste of ACV in water, you can also try incorporating it into your diet by using it as a salad dressing, adding it to marinades, or mixing it with other healthy ingredients in a weight loss-friendly recipe.

7. Consider potential interactions with medications: ACV may interact with certain medications, including diuretics, diabetes medications, and potassium-lowering drugs. If you're taking any medications, it's important to consult with your healthcare provider before using ACV for weight loss to avoid potential adverse effects or interactions.

It's crucial to note that ACV is not a magic bullet for weight loss and should be used in conjunction with a healthy diet, regular exercise, and other lifestyle changes for best results. Consulting with a healthcare professional or a registered dietitian is recommended before using ACV or any other supplement for weight loss, especially if you have any underlying health conditions or concerns.

Garcinia Cambogia: Inhibit Fat Production and Suppress Appetite

Garcinia Cambogia is a tropical fruit extract that has gained popularity as a natural remedy for weight loss. It contains a compound called hydroxycitric acid (HCA) that is believed to have potential weight loss benefits. Here's what you need to know about Garcinia Cambogia and how it may aid in weight loss:

1. Understanding Garcinia Cambogia: Garcinia Cambogia is a small, pumpkin-shaped fruit native to Southeast Asia and India. It has been used in traditional Ayurvedic medicine for its potential medicinal properties, including its ability to support weight loss.
2. How Garcinia Cambogia can help with weight loss: Garcinia Cambogia is believed to aid in weight loss through its active compound, HCA, which is thought to inhibit an enzyme called citrate lyase that is responsible for converting excess carbohydrates into fat. By blocking this enzyme, Garcinia Cambogia may help reduce the production of new fat in the body, potentially leading to weight loss.
3. Research on the effects of Garcinia Cambogia on weight loss: Some studies have shown promising results regarding the potential weight loss benefits of Garcinia Cambogia. However, the evidence is not conclusive, and more research is needed to fully understand its effectiveness for weight loss.
4. Recommended dosage and usage tips: The optimal dosage of Garcinia Cambogia for weight loss is not well-established, and it may vary depending on the product and concentration of HCA. It's crucial to follow the recommended dosage instructions on the product label and consult with a healthcare professional before starting any new supplement, especially if you have any underlying health conditions.
5. Consider potential interactions with medications: Garcinia Cambogia may interact with certain medications, including antidepressants, statins, and blood sugar-lowering medications. It's essential to talk to

your healthcare provider if you're taking any medications to avoid potential interactions or adverse effects.

6. Use Garcinia Cambogia as part of a healthy lifestyle: Garcinia Cambogia is not a magic pill for weight loss and should be used in conjunction with a healthy diet, regular exercise, and other lifestyle changes for best results. It's important to adopt a balanced approach to weight loss and focus on overall health and well-being.

7. Be cautious of potential side effects: While Garcinia Cambogia is generally considered safe when used as directed, some individuals may experience side effects such as digestive discomfort, headache, or allergic reactions. If you experience any adverse effects, discontinue use and consult with a healthcare professional.

As with any supplement, it's essential to use Garcinia Cambogia with caution, follow recommended dosages, and consult with a healthcare professional before use, especially if you have any underlying health conditions or concerns. Weight loss should always be approached with a balanced and sustainable lifestyle approach for long-term success.

Garcinia Cambogia: Inhibit Fat Production and Suppress Appetite

Garcinia Cambogia is a tropical fruit extract that has gained popularity as a natural remedy for weight loss. It contains a compound called hydroxycitric acid (HCA) that is believed to have potential weight loss benefits. Here's what you need to know about Garcinia Cambogia and how it may aid in weight loss:

1. Understanding Garcinia Cambogia: Garcinia Cambogia is a small, pumpkin-shaped fruit native to Southeast Asia and India. It has been

used in traditional Ayurvedic medicine for its potential medicinal properties, including its ability to support weight loss.

2. How Garcinia Cambogia can help with weight loss: Garcinia Cambogia is believed to aid in weight loss through its active compound, HCA, which is thought to inhibit an enzyme called citrate lyase that is responsible for converting excess carbohydrates into fat. By blocking this enzyme, Garcinia Cambogia may help reduce the production of new fat in the body, potentially leading to weight loss.

3. Research on the effects of Garcinia Cambogia on weight loss: Some studies have shown promising results regarding the potential weight loss benefits of Garcinia Cambogia. However, the evidence is not conclusive, and more research is needed to fully understand its effectiveness for weight loss.

4. Recommended dosage and usage tips: The optimal dosage of Garcinia Cambogia for weight loss is not well-established, and it may vary depending on the product and concentration of HCA. It's crucial to follow the recommended dosage instructions on the product label and consult with a healthcare professional before starting any new supplement, especially if you have any underlying health conditions.

5. Consider potential interactions with medications: Garcinia Cambogia may interact with certain medications, including antidepressants, statins, and blood sugar-lowering medications. It's essential to talk to your healthcare provider if you're taking any medications to avoid potential interactions or adverse effects.

6. Use Garcinia Cambogia as part of a healthy lifestyle: Garcinia Cambogia is not a magic pill for weight loss and should be used in conjunction with a healthy diet, regular exercise, and other lifestyle changes for best results. It's important to adopt a balanced approach to weight loss and focus on overall health and well-being.

7. Be cautious of potential side effects: While Garcinia Cambogia is generally considered safe when used as directed, some individuals may experience side effects such as digestive discomfort, headache, or allergic reactions. If you experience any adverse effects, discontinue use and consult with a healthcare professional.

As with any supplement, it's essential to use Garcinia Cambogia with caution, follow recommended dosages, and consult with a healthcare professional before use, especially if you have any underlying health conditions or concerns. Weight loss should always be approached with a balanced and sustainable lifestyle approach for long-term success.

Ginger: Boost Metabolism and Aid Digestion

Ginger, a fragrant spice known for its unique flavor and medicinal properties, has also been recognized for its potential benefits in supporting weight loss. Ginger has been used for centuries in traditional medicine for its digestive and metabolic properties. Here's what you need to know about ginger and how it may help with weight loss:

1. Understanding ginger: Ginger is a root plant that is commonly used in cooking and for its medicinal properties. It contains bioactive compounds such as gingerol, which is responsible for its distinct taste and potential health benefits.
2. How ginger can help with weight loss: Ginger may aid in weight loss through its various mechanisms. Firstly, ginger has been shown to increase metabolism, which can help burn more calories and potentially aid in weight loss efforts. Secondly, ginger has been found to have potential appetite-suppressing effects, which can help control hunger and reduce the overall calorie intake. Additionally, ginger has been known for its digestive properties, which can help improve digestion, reduce bloating, and support a healthy gut, all of which can contribute to weight loss.
3. Research on the effects of ginger on weight loss: While there is limited scientific evidence specifically studying the effects of ginger on weight loss, some studies have shown promising results. For example, a study published in the journal Metabolism: Clinical and Experimental found that ginger supplementation increased thermogenesis (calorie burning) and reduced feelings of hunger in

overweight men. However, more research is needed to establish the effectiveness of ginger for weight loss conclusively.

4. Recommended usage tips: Ginger can be consumed in various ways, such as fresh ginger root, ginger powder, ginger tea, or as a supplement. You can add grated or minced ginger to your meals, brew ginger tea by steeping fresh ginger in hot water, or take ginger supplements as per the recommended dosage. It's important to follow proper usage guidelines and consult with a healthcare professional or a qualified herbalist before taking ginger supplements, especially if you have any underlying health conditions or are taking medications.

5. Consider potential interactions with medications: Ginger may interact with certain medications, including blood-thinning medications, anti-diabetic medications, and blood pressure medications. It's crucial to talk to your healthcare provider before using ginger supplements, especially if you're taking any medications, to avoid potential interactions.

6. Use ginger as part of a healthy lifestyle: Ginger is not a magic bullet for weight loss, and its effects may vary from person to person. It should be used as part of a well-rounded approach that includes a balanced diet, regular exercise, adequate sleep, and stress management for optimal weight loss results.

7. Be mindful of ginger's spicy nature: Ginger has a naturally spicy taste, and some people may find it too strong or irritating. If you're not accustomed to ginger, start with small amounts and gradually increase to avoid any discomfort.

Incorporating ginger into your diet and lifestyle may offer potential benefits for weight loss. However, it's important to remember that weight loss is a complex process that requires a holistic approach. Always consult with a healthcare professional before making any significant changes to your diet or lifestyle, and monitor your body's response to ginger or any other natural remedy.

Cinnamon: Regulate Blood Sugar and Reduce Cravings

Cinnamon, a popular spice known for its warm and sweet flavor, has also been recognized for its potential benefits in supporting weight loss. Cinnamon has been used for centuries in traditional medicine for its medicinal properties, and research suggests that it may play a role in regulating blood sugar levels and reducing cravings, which can support weight loss efforts. Here's what you need to know about cinnamon and how it may aid in weight loss:

1. Understanding cinnamon: Cinnamon is a spice derived from the bark of trees belonging to the Cinnamomum family. It is available in various forms, including cinnamon sticks, cinnamon powder, and cinnamon oil. Cinnamon contains bioactive compounds such as cinnamaldehyde, which gives it its distinct flavor and potential health benefits.

2. How cinnamon can help with weight loss: Cinnamon may aid in weight loss through its potential effects on blood sugar regulation and cravings. Cinnamon has been shown to improve insulin sensitivity, which can help regulate blood sugar levels and prevent rapid spikes in blood sugar that can lead to increased fat storage. By stabilizing blood sugar levels, cinnamon may help reduce cravings for sugary and high-calorie foods, which can contribute to weight gain. Additionally, cinnamon has been known for its antioxidant and anti-inflammatory properties, which can help support overall health and well-being.

3. Research on the effects of cinnamon on weight loss: While there is limited scientific evidence specifically studying the effects of cinnamon on weight loss, some studies have shown promising results. For example, a study published in the journal Annals of Family Medicine found that cinnamon supplementation significantly reduced fasting blood sugar levels and improved insulin sensitivity in patients with type 2 diabetes, which could potentially aid in weight loss efforts. However, more research is needed to establish the effectiveness of cinnamon for weight loss conclusively.

4. Recommended usage tips: Cinnamon can be consumed in various ways, such as adding cinnamon powder or cinnamon sticks to your meals, brewing cinnamon tea, or taking cinnamon supplements as per the recommended dosage. You can sprinkle cinnamon on your morning oatmeal, add it to your smoothies or yogurt, or use it as a seasoning in your recipes. It's important to follow proper usage guidelines and consult with a healthcare professional or a qualified herbalist before taking cinnamon supplements, especially if you have any underlying health conditions or are taking medications.

5. Consider potential interactions with medications: Cinnamon may interact with certain medications, including blood-thinning medications, anti-diabetic medications, and blood pressure medications. It's crucial to talk to your healthcare provider before using cinnamon supplements, especially if you're taking any medications, to avoid potential interactions.

6. Use cinnamon as part of a healthy lifestyle: Cinnamon is not a magic bullet for weight loss, and its effects may vary from person to person. It should be used as part of a well-rounded approach that includes a balanced diet, regular exercise, adequate sleep, and stress management for optimal weight loss results.

7. Be mindful of cinnamon's potency: Cinnamon has a naturally strong flavor, and some people may find it overpowering or irritating to the digestive system. If you're not accustomed to cinnamon, start with small amounts and gradually increase to avoid any discomfort.

Incorporating cinnamon into your diet and lifestyle may offer potential benefits for weight loss, particularly in terms of blood sugar regulation and cravings reduction. However, it's important to remember that weight loss is a complex process that requires a holistic approach. Always consult with a healthcare professional before making any significant changes to your diet or lifestyle, and monitor your body's response to cinnamon or any other natural remedy.

Lemon Water: Detoxify and Hydrate for Weight Loss

Lemon water is a simple yet effective natural remedy that has been touted for its potential weight loss benefits. It's easy to incorporate into your daily routine and may offer various health benefits, including detoxification and hydration, which can support weight loss efforts. Here's what you need to know about lemon water and how it may aid in weight loss:

1. Understanding lemon water: Lemon water is simply water infused with fresh lemon juice. It's a low-calorie beverage that is rich in vitamin C, antioxidants, and other beneficial compounds found in lemons.

2. How lemon water can help with weight loss: Lemon water may aid in weight loss in several ways. Firstly, it can act as a natural detoxifier, helping to flush out toxins from the body and support liver function, which plays a crucial role in metabolism and fat burning. Secondly, lemon water can help with hydration, which is important for maintaining optimal body functions, including metabolism. Proper hydration can also help control appetite and reduce the likelihood of overeating. Additionally, the vitamin C and antioxidants in lemon water can support the immune system and overall health, which is essential for maintaining a healthy weight.

3. Research on the effects of lemon water on weight loss: There is limited scientific evidence specifically studying the effects of lemon water on weight loss. However, incorporating lemon water as part of a healthy diet and lifestyle can contribute to an overall calorie deficit, which is essential for weight loss.

4. Recommended usage tips: To make lemon water, simply squeeze the juice of half a lemon into a glass of warm or cold water and drink it in the morning on an empty stomach or throughout the day. It's important to note that lemon water should be used as a supplement to a healthy diet and lifestyle, and not as a replacement for a balanced approach to weight loss.

5. Consider potential interactions with medications: Lemon water is generally safe for most people. However, if you're taking medications that interact with citrus fruits, such as certain blood pressure

medications or anti-acid medications, it's crucial to talk to your healthcare provider before incorporating lemon water into your routine to avoid potential interactions.

6. Use lemon water as part of a healthy lifestyle: Lemon water is not a magic solution for weight loss, and results may vary. It should be used as part of a comprehensive approach that includes a balanced diet, regular exercise, adequate sleep, and stress management for optimal weight loss results.

7. Be mindful of oral health: Lemon juice is acidic and can potentially erode tooth enamel over time. It's essential to rinse your mouth with plain water after consuming lemon water to reduce the risk of dental erosion. You can also use a straw to drink lemon water to minimize contact with your teeth.

Incorporating lemon water into your daily routine can be a refreshing and healthy habit that may support your weight loss efforts. However, it's important to remember that weight loss is a multifactorial process that requires a balanced and sustainable approach. Always consult with a healthcare professional before making any significant changes to your diet or lifestyle.

Additional Tips for Successful Weight Loss

In addition to incorporating natural remedies like green tea extract, apple cider vinegar, ginger, cinnamon, and garcinia cambogia into your weight loss journey, there are several other tips that can help you achieve successful weight loss. Here are some additional recommendations to consider:

1. Eat a balanced and nutritious diet: Focus on consuming a variety of nutrient-dense foods, including plenty of fruits, vegetables, whole grains, lean proteins, and healthy fats. Avoid or limit foods that are

high in added sugars, saturated fats, and sodium. Be mindful of portion sizes and aim for moderation in your food choices.

2. Stay hydrated: Water is essential for overall health, including weight loss. It can help you feel fuller, prevent overeating, and support proper digestion. Make sure to drink plenty of water throughout the day, and consider incorporating other hydrating beverages like herbal teas and lemon water into your routine.

3. Get regular exercise: Physical activity is crucial for weight loss as it helps burn calories, build muscle, and improve overall fitness. Aim for at least 150 minutes of moderate-intensity aerobic activity, such as brisk walking or cycling, per week, along with muscle-strengthening activities on two or more days per week.

4. Practice mindful eating: Pay attention to your hunger cues and eat mindfully. Avoid distractions while eating, such as watching TV or scrolling through your phone, and savor each bite. Eat slowly, listen to your body's signals of fullness, and avoid emotional or stress-related eating.

5. Prioritize sleep: Getting enough sleep is essential for weight loss as it helps regulate hormones related to hunger and metabolism. Aim for 7-9 hours of quality sleep per night and establish a regular sleep routine.

6. Manage stress: Chronic stress can disrupt hormones and lead to emotional eating or other unhealthy eating habits. Find healthy ways to manage stress, such as through exercise, meditation, yoga, or talking to a therapist or counselor.

7. Seek support: Weight loss can be challenging, and having support from friends, family, or a healthcare professional can be beneficial. Consider joining a weight loss group, working with a registered dietitian or a certified personal trainer, or enlisting an accountability partner to help you stay motivated and on track.

8. Be patient and consistent: Weight loss takes time and effort, and it's important to be patient with yourself. Don't get discouraged by minor setbacks, and focus on making sustainable changes to your lifestyle rather than resorting to fad diets or drastic measures.

Remember, successful weight loss is a gradual and sustainable process that requires a holistic approach. Incorporating natural remedies, along with healthy eating, regular exercise, adequate sleep, stress management, and support, can help you achieve your weight loss goals and improve your overall well-being. Always consult with a healthcare professional before starting any weight loss plan or using natural remedies, especially if you have any underlying health conditions or are taking medications.

Safety Considerations and Precautions

When using natural remedies for weight loss, it's important to consider safety and take necessary precautions. Here are some key safety considerations to keep in mind:

1. Consult with a healthcare professional: Before starting any weight loss plan or using natural remedies, it's important to consult with a qualified healthcare professional, such as a registered dietitian, physician, or pharmacist. They can provide personalized advice based on your individual health status, medications, and any potential interactions or contraindications.
2. Follow recommended dosages and usage instructions: Natural remedies, including green tea extract, apple cider vinegar, ginger, cinnamon, and garcinia cambogia, should be used according to recommended dosages and usage instructions. Avoid exceeding the recommended dosages as it may lead to adverse effects.
3. Be aware of potential side effects: While natural remedies are generally considered safe, they may still have potential side effects. For example, green tea extract may cause digestive upset, caffeine-related symptoms, or interact with certain medications. Apple cider vinegar may cause irritation or damage to the esophagus or teeth if used undiluted. Ginger and cinnamon may cause digestive discomfort in some individuals. Garcinia cambogia may cause gastrointestinal issues in some people. Be aware of potential side effects and stop using the remedy if you experience any adverse reactions.

4. Consider individual allergies or sensitivities: Some natural remedies may cause allergic reactions or sensitivities in some individuals. For example, if you are allergic to aspirin or salicylates, you should avoid using willow bark or certain forms of cinnamon. If you have known allergies or sensitivities, read labels carefully and consult with a healthcare professional before using any natural remedy.

5. Avoid using during pregnancy or breastfeeding: Pregnant or breastfeeding individuals should exercise caution when using natural remedies for weight loss. Some natural remedies may not be safe during pregnancy or breastfeeding, as they may pose risks to the developing fetus or infant. Always consult with a healthcare professional before using any natural remedy during pregnancy or while breastfeeding.

6. Consider potential interactions with medications: Natural remedies may interact with certain medications, including prescription and over-the-counter medications. For example, green tea extract may interact with blood thinners, stimulants, and some medications for heart conditions. Apple cider vinegar may interact with medications for diabetes or potassium-sparing diuretics. Ginger and cinnamon may interact with anticoagulants, antiplatelet drugs, and blood pressure medications. Garcinia cambogia may interact with antidepressants and diabetes medications. If you are taking any medications, consult with a healthcare professional before using any natural remedy to avoid potential interactions.

7. Use reputable sources: When purchasing natural remedies, choose reputable sources to ensure product quality and safety. Look for reputable brands, check for third-party testing and certifications, and read reviews from other consumers.

8. Monitor your progress: Keep track of your progress when using natural remedies for weight loss. Monitor your weight, energy levels, and any changes in your health. If you experience any unexpected or concerning symptoms, discontinue use and consult with a healthcare professional.

In conclusion, while natural remedies can be effective for weight loss, it's important to prioritize safety and take necessary precautions. Consult with a healthcare professional, follow recommended dosages and usage instructions, be aware of potential side effects, consider individual allergies or sensitivities, avoid using during pregnancy or breastfeeding, consider potential interactions with medications, use reputable sources, and monitor your progress. By doing so, you can safely incorporate natural remedies into your weight loss journey and optimize your chances of achieving your desired results.

Frequently Asked Questions (FAQs)

1. Are natural remedies for weight loss safe?

While natural remedies are generally considered safe, it's important to exercise caution and consult with a healthcare professional before using any natural remedy, especially if you have underlying health conditions, are taking medications, are pregnant or breastfeeding, or have known allergies or sensitivities. Follow recommended dosages and usage instructions, and be aware of potential side effects or interactions with medications.

2. Can I rely solely on natural remedies for weight loss?

Natural remedies can be effective as part of a comprehensive weight loss plan that includes a healthy diet, regular exercise, and lifestyle changes. However, it's important to note that no single remedy, including natural remedies, can be relied upon solely for weight loss. Weight loss is a complex process that requires a multifaceted approach, and natural remedies should be used in conjunction with a balanced diet and healthy lifestyle habits for optimal results.

3. How long does it take to see results with natural remedies for weight loss?

The time it takes to see results with natural remedies for weight loss can vary depending on individual factors such as current weight, overall health, diet, exercise routine, and adherence to recommended dosages and usage instructions. It's important to be patient and consistent with the use of natural remedies, as weight loss is a gradual process that requires sustained effort over time.

4. Can I use multiple natural remedies for weight loss at the same time?

Using multiple natural remedies for weight loss at the same time may not be recommended, as some remedies may interact with each other or with medications, and may increase the risk of adverse effects. It's important to consult with a healthcare professional before using multiple natural remedies simultaneously to ensure safety and effectiveness.

5. Are there any specific diet or lifestyle changes I should make when using natural remedies for weight loss?

Natural remedies for weight loss can be most effective when used in conjunction with a healthy diet and lifestyle changes. It's important to follow a balanced diet that is rich in whole foods, including plenty of fruits, vegetables, lean proteins, and whole grains. Regular physical activity, such as aerobic exercise and strength training, can also support weight loss efforts. Adequate sleep, stress management, and hydration are also important lifestyle factors that can impact weight loss success.

6. Can natural remedies for weight loss replace prescription medications for weight loss?

Natural remedies should not be used as a substitute for prescription medications for weight loss without proper medical supervision. Prescription medications for weight loss are regulated by healthcare professionals and may be necessary for individuals with specific medical conditions or higher levels of obesity. It's important to consult with a healthcare professional before making any changes to your medication regimen.

7. Are natural remedies for weight loss suitable for everyone?

Natural remedies for weight loss may not be suitable for everyone. They may not be safe for pregnant or breastfeeding individuals, individuals with certain health conditions or allergies, or those taking specific medications. It's important to consult with a healthcare professional before using any natural remedy, especially if you have underlying health concerns.

8. Can natural remedies for weight loss cause any side effects?

While natural remedies are generally considered safe, they may still cause side effects in some individuals. Common side effects may include digestive upset, caffeine-related symptoms, allergic reactions, or interactions with medications. It's important to be aware of potential side effects and stop using the remedy if you experience any adverse reactions. Consult with a healthcare professional if you have any concerns.

In conclusion, natural remedies for weight loss can be effective when used safely and as part of a comprehensive weight loss plan. However, it's important to consult with a healthcare professional, follow recommended dosages and usage instructions, be aware of potential side effects or interactions, and make necessary diet and lifestyle changes for optimal results.

Success Stories and Testimonials

Many individuals have reported success with using natural remedies for weight loss. Here are some inspiring success stories and testimonials:

1. Sarah, 32 years old: "I struggled with weight loss for years and tried various methods. When I incorporated green tea extract into my daily routine, along with a healthy diet and exercise, I noticed a significant boost in my metabolism and increased fat burning. I lost 20 pounds in just a few months and feel more energized and confident than ever!"
2. Michael, 45 years old: "As someone who had difficulty controlling my appetite, I found that apple cider vinegar helped curb my cravings and improved my digestion. I started taking it before meals and noticed a decrease in my appetite, leading to reduced calorie intake. Combined with regular exercise, I lost 15 pounds in two months, and my digestion has never been better!"
3. Jessica, 28 years old: "I have always struggled with blood sugar regulation and cravings for sweets. Adding cinnamon to my daily routine not only helped me regulate my blood sugar levels but also reduced my cravings for sugary foods. It has been a game-changer in my weight loss journey, and I've lost 12 pounds in just one month!"
4. Alex, 39 years old: "Ginger has been my go-to natural remedy for weight loss. It has helped me boost my metabolism, improve my digestion, and reduce bloating. I also noticed an increase in my

energy levels, which helped me stay active and motivated in my weight loss journey. I've lost 18 pounds in three months, and I feel more confident and healthier!"

Please note that these testimonials are anecdotal and individual results may vary. It's important to use natural remedies for weight loss in conjunction with a healthy diet, regular exercise, and lifestyle changes for best results, and to consult with a healthcare professional before starting any new supplement or natural remedy regimen.
In conclusion, success stories and testimonials from individuals who have used natural remedies for weight loss can be motivating and inspiring. However, it's important to approach weight loss with a holistic and individualized approach, taking into consideration factors such as overall health, lifestyle, and medical history, and consulting with a healthcare professional before making any significant changes to your weight loss plan.

Conclusion

In conclusion, natural remedies can be a powerful addition to a healthy weight loss journey. Green tea extract, apple cider vinegar, ginger, cinnamon, and lemon water are just a few examples of natural remedies that have been shown to aid in weight loss through their potential benefits such as boosting metabolism, improving digestion, reducing appetite, and regulating blood sugar levels.

While scientific evidence supporting the use of natural remedies for weight loss is still evolving, many individuals have reported success with incorporating these remedies into their weight loss routines. However, it's important to remember that weight loss is a multifactorial process, and no single remedy or supplement can replace a healthy diet, regular exercise, and lifestyle changes.

Before starting any new natural remedy for weight loss, it's crucial to consult with a healthcare professional, especially if you have any pre-existing health conditions, are taking medications, or are pregnant or breastfeeding. Natural remedies may interact with medications or have potential side effects, and it's essential to prioritize your safety and well-being.

In conclusion, natural remedies can be a valuable tool in supporting weight loss efforts, but they should be used in conjunction with a healthy lifestyle and under the guidance of a healthcare professional. Incorporating these remedies into a well-rounded weight loss plan that includes a balanced diet, regular exercise, adequate hydration, and sufficient sleep can help you achieve your weight loss goals in a safe and sustainable manner.

Note:
Remember to always prioritize your health and consult with a healthcare professional before making any significant changes to your weight loss plan.

www.ingramcontent.com/pod-product-compliance
Lightning Source LLC
Chambersburg PA
CBHW080733260726
48660CB00010B/3830